Table of contents:

Ch1. Why Approaching Is So Scary

It's Saturday and you're out. People are walking by as you make your way forward, lost to the world or daydreaming about meeting with your friends tonight. That's when you see her, a complete smoking bombshell of a girl just getting out of her car. Everything slows as you hyper focus on her, noticing the shine of her lip gloss and how her shirt doesn't fully cover her waist.

This hyper awareness continues as she starts walking...directly toward you. Immediately you begin wishing you could say something, anything, to get her attention and meet this divine angel. That's when the anxiety hits though. Worst case scenarios of her looking at you in disgust flash across your mind, of everyone around you laughing at your attempt. Hell, why would a girl like THAT even want to talk to you?

"She's probably busy or in a rush," you tell yourself. "I bet she has a boyfriend," may be another thought. She finally walks past without you saying a word, and you sigh in relief. "Only creepy guys approach random women anyway," you finally conclude. Just like that, you've once again thrown away the perfect chance to meet the kind of girl you truly desire. Approach anxiety strikes again!

Why God, why?!

Unfortunately this scenario is so common among men that I'm sure every single person reading this has experienced that scenario (or one just like it), not just once, but several times...this month.

It's sad, but on average, the typical man will only approach 10 women in his lifetime. *That's it.* To make matters worse, almost all of those approaches will usually end up nowhere. Yet even this number is misleading due to the 80/20 rule, which states that only 20% of the male population is REALLY doing the approaching. I myself have approached in the thousands range, if not 10,000 women, which vastly skews the average. I'd guess that the real average guy approaches maybe twice in his life...if at all.

Thankfully, most men don't need to, though. Instead, they prefer meeting girls in class, at work, through friends, or using online dating sites like Tinder. While this is fine for most, it still leads to massive opportunities lost for meeting incredible women in person. Once a guy can master the art of the approach, something miraculous happens as well...it becomes FUN. All the approach anxiety turns into approach excitement! Sure there's always a little bit of unease, but the thrill and excitement of meeting a girl you're attracted to right there on the spot is unlike anything else you'll ever feel. To do this, though, you must understand where this fear comes from.

The first reason is just the way we're all wired through thousands of years of evolution. While we can enjoy a never ending stream of women to meet due to the population size, this wasn't always the case. Back in caveman times, we only came into contact with a very small sample size of women. If one of our ancestors approached the wrong woman, he may have been clubbed to death by her partner, or have started a war with another village! Even if she wasn't already taken, the failure of such an approach could leave him shamed, as the woman would spread news of his feeble attempt to all the other women in the village. Just like that, his entire pool of women to choose from in the WORLD would be gone. It's no wonder our ancestors were the ones who played things a little more safe.

Society has another huge role in this, as well. Outside of a James Bond movie, approaching random women doesn't exactly have the best connotation, now does it? We often see these guys as players, who are shallow, or desperate at best. At worst? Well, we're now talking about creeps, pervs, and degenerates. Not exactly the best image to have of yourself. But in the words of **Hitch**, "No girl wakes up hoping she doesn't randomly meet the guy of her dreams."

Thankfully, society's views are slowly changing, and it's acknowledging the courage and confidence it takes to approach a girl. It's now seen as highly impressive and awe inspiring to tell your friends you just met your girlfriend while walking down the street one day. It's my hope this trend will continue, and that if you're reading this book, you'll also be able to gain a sense of pride from mastering this rare ability.

Another issue we face that causes approach anxiety is our conditioning. From a young age we've been told never to go and talk to strangers. What's worse is that during their puberty years, boys and girls sit at separate tables and form cliques of the same gender. God forbid a boy tries to make a flirtatious attempt with a girl out of the blue. Unless he's already seen as popular, it's almost always a harsh rejection. This can be some of the most embarrassing moments in our lives and shape who we eventually become.

I still vividly remember asking a girl out, who laughed and told me no. Within a few hours every girl in class was coming up to me asking, "Did you REALLY just ask out Amanda?!". Within one day I completely destroyed my dating pool. It seems the cavemen were right (when it comes to high school at least).

With all this said, you know the REAL reason why guys don't approach? The number one thing holding them back?

Approaching attractive women is just not part of their identity.

It really is that simple. As Aristotle once said, "We are what we repeatedly do." Every time you see a beautiful girl walk by and you don't approach, you're telling yourself, "Yup, I'm a guy who doesn't approach women I find attractive." The more this goes on, the harder and harder it becomes to break the identity.

Easily the toughest and most stubborn students I get when coaching are the ones over 40. By the time a man has gotten to that age, they're just set in their ways. This doesn't mean a guy can't change. I have countless success stories for older men. One of my older students allowed me to be there when he proposed to his girlfriend (one he met from a cold approach) and later, invited me to his wedding. So if you're reading this and you're over 40, don't worry, everything in this book will work for you as well. If you have an open mind, that is.

Staying true to one's identity, and ideally changing it if needed, is one of the single hardest things a man can do. I'll almost certainly cover this in another book since this topic really deserves its own, but for now, I'll explain the basics as it relates to approaching

The logical levels of change is a Neuro Linguistic Programing idea (NLP for short) proposed by Robert Dilts and Todd Epstein. Here's what it looks like.

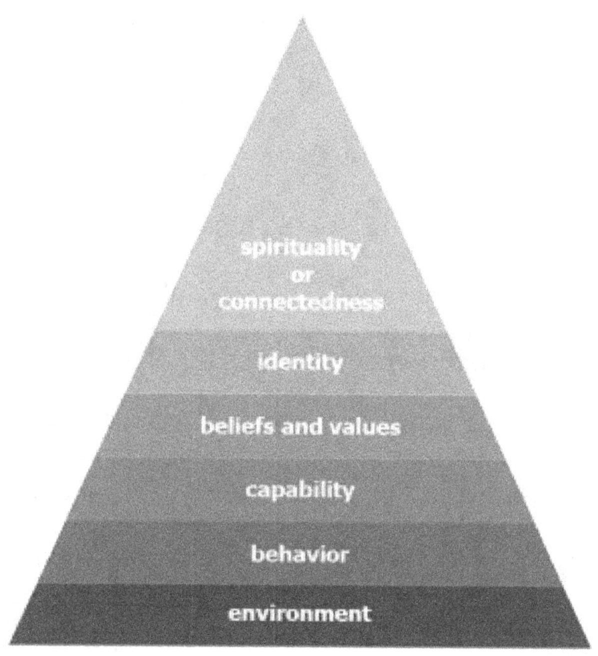

The easiest level to change is one's environment, followed then by one's behavior and so on. The hardest levels are the top ones being a person's spiritual connectedness and, surprise surprise, one's

identity. The good news is you can work on all the levels at once. I'll even be giving you numerous tips in this book on how to do that. What's even better is, if you master one of the higher levels, the lower ones tend to begin changing on their own.

These levels interfere on every aspect before we ever approach a girl. Let's take the following sentence as an example:

"I can't approach her here."

I'm sure every guy reading this has had this thought pop up at one time or another. If we break down this thought word by word though, we realize how every level plays a part. Note that the spiritual level of change is a man's purpose or meaning in life. The idea that this thought exists at all shows the spiritual level.

"**I** can't approach her here." - Emphasis on the **identity** level: Who could do it if not you? What can you do?

"I **can't** approach her here." - Emphasis on the **beliefs and values** level: What's stopping me from doing the approach? Who or what says I can't do it?

"I can't **approach** her here." - Emphasis on the **capability** level: Do I need a special skill set for this? Is there a method I don't know?

"I can't approach **her** here." - Emphasis on the **behavior** level: Do you have positive intentions for her? What kind of actions do you need for her? Are the actions you need in accordance to your personal development?

"I can't approach her **here.**" - Emphasis on the **environment** level: Where and when can you approach? What is the ideal approach environment? What time of day or night is best?

All of these questions must be asked when thoughts like this pop up. Instead of taking the thought at face value, we need to understand it all comes from a negative identity towards approaching women.

At your core, you are a learning machine. Unfortunately if you learn something negative and let it grow, it can infect you the same way a virus can infect a computer. It's my hope that by reading this book and questioning your current beliefs, we can reprogram your machine so it's operating at its finest level. If you haven't already I highly recommend reading the book "Psycho-cybernetics" by Maxwell Maltz, who goes into this topic in incredible detail. It's basically required reading for my students and more than one has reported to me that they began crying when reading the powerful messages that book has to offer.

Now that you know WHY you have approach anxiety we can finally get into the real reason you bought this book, which is HOW to overcome it. I explain the "why" though to emphasize two key things. First, there are numerous things working against you mastering this skill, there's no easy fix and like anything, it will require practice and patience.

The second reason is that I truly believe that only by understanding where this stems from can you confront it head on. You don't need to blindly follow my suggestions but instead can see the truth of things for yourself. Now that you're ready, let's learn how to get rid of that pesky anxiety for good.

Ch. 2 How To Get Over The Fear

Approach anxiety, social anxiety, panic attacks, hell even something called Generalized Anxiety Disorder (GAD) run rampant amongst the population. Now I'm not saying everyone has some form of anxiety disorder, but other than depression, it's easily the most common problem therapists see.

When talking about fear and anxiety, we need to understand it's a spectrum. The anxiety can be really high or it can be really low, but it's never gone completely. As I stated earlier, I've approached around 10,000 women and I can assure you I had some level of anxiety for every single one. It's not like a light switch to just turn off. Real mastery is learning how to feel the anxiety **and approach anyways**.

Why am I telling you this? Because too many guys use the excuse of having any anxiety as the rationale for why they can't approach. They'll use the techniques I'm about to teach you and instead of controlling their anxiety and approaching anyway, they keep doing exercises in the hopes that they will get into a "state" where they feel no anxiety. This idea of getting into state is similar to an athlete being in the zone. Often, Lebron James will get momentum going in a basketball game and he'll seem to be on fire, just making every shot and performing at an insane level. This is great and is true for approaching, as well. It doesn't mean you DEPEND on it though.

The first, and arguably best trick to "getting in state" and making approaching feel easier is...well...approaching. Not what you expected or wanted to be told, I know, but hear me out. The first approach may be terrifying and rough, maybe even the second one too. Usually though, something magical happens after we do a few approaches where they continue to progressively become easier. All of a sudden "one more approach" doesn't seem as big a deal. Hell, you were wondering why you were making such a big deal about it in the first place.

Remember how I talked about conditioning being one of the reasons guys don't approach? Most guys may get the courage to do one approach and experience the fear of doing it, followed by (most likely) a rejection from the girl. Well after getting punished like that, NO WONDER they don't want to try it again. Yet for the few brave at heart who keep doing it, one right after another, they experience what I'm talking about and usually get into state. Ah, the miracle of systematic desensitization at work.

Systematic desensitization was discovered by South African psychiatrist Joseph Wolpe in 1958. He found that by gradually introducing an object that causes anxiety to a patient, the patient would eventually be able to lower their anxiety until it was no longer a problem. Based on his work, this process occurs in three steps.

The first step is identifying an anxiety hierarchy. For our purposes, we'll obviously use the example of approaching a girl. Think of the scariest approach possible. Maybe it involves a gorgeous model surrounded by guy and girl friends in a large group, who happens to have a resting bitch face. Now think of the easiest approach. This one may involve a single girl, who looks cute and inviting, in a place you feel comfortable at, with few people around. Now think of several other scenarios in between, and rank them from least to most scary. The idea here is to start small for practice and gradually push yourself to do harder scenarios.

Going into the second step is about learning the correct response. **The most important thing is to relax**. Don't worry if she likes you or saying something cool; not at first. When you first begin going out to try and approach women you like, you HAVE to see it as practice. When going up, give yourself permission to fail. Hell, expect it even. Once again this is practice and has no real consequences for you. Remind yourself that you'll never see this girl again, and that ultimately, this one approach doesn't matter, but your development does. The initial goal is to challenge yourself in seeing how comfortable you can possibly be with every approach that you do.

The third step is simple: you listen to Nike and "just do it." With your goal of relaxing in mind, as well as the mentality that it's all just for practice, you can gradually increase the difficulty of each approach. At first, you may just do a functional opener (discussed later in this book) by saying something like, "Excuse me could you give me directions to X street?" Maybe you ask for her name but then leave after that. It's OK! The goal, though, is for every approach to be a little more intimate/flirty and to last longer. I've told my students repeatedly that you "need to allow yourself to be garbage now to become a legend later."

So you're going out knowing it's all for practice and you're just meant to relax as you try this out, yet you're still incredibly uncomfortable. Well tough luck, you need to get comfortable with being uncomfortable. There's a reason the vast majority of guys aren't able to do this; it's seriously tough! Luckily you're not the kind of guy that will easily quit, right? Good, I didn't think so. It's important to set your expectations correctly, because while you're relaxed reading this, you may feel pumped up and wanting to try it out. Yet the moment you find a girl and think about approaching, that fear comes shooting right back. This is what you need to prepare for, and more importantly, EXPECT.

The good news is that you don't need to be out approaching to do systematic desensitization. Yes, you read that correctly. Instead you can use a technique called "creative visualization" that's been used as early as the ancient Greek days. In the 70's and 80's, numerous psychologists began realizing that this technique was also incredibly powerful for dealing with anxiety, as well. The idea is when you're home alone, imagine, in as much detail as possible, the approach scenario. What do you see, hear, smell? Run this "simulation" through your mind's eye and see yourself approaching the girl. Maybe the girl is really receptive and interested in you right away. Then again, maybe she rejects you on the spot, but you visualize how you don't lose your composure, and it has no effect on you. While it will never replace the real thing, this exercise will add to you becoming desensitized to the approach. Go ahead and try it now a few times, before reading on.

I would do this religiously, both the actual practice of approaching and the visualization. When I first started, I'd go and approach anywhere between 10-30 girls, 6 times a week. You could say I was a bit obsessed trying to figure this out! I'd also do these visualizations every night before bed and every morning when I woke up. Within a couple of months, I could already see not just my approach getting better, but how I felt, as well.

To this day, I still vividly remember one approach where, for some reason, the nerves just took hold of my entire body. I walked up to her and just spat out nonsensical verbal diarrhea. It went something like this:

Me: "Hey, I just wanted to, you know, get your opinion about something that I...because if you think about it then... maybe you could help me with this thing, but I don't know, can you?"

This sweet girl kindly just looked at me, smiling, and asked, "What was that?" before I once again said a bunch of nonsense back to her. After she walked off, though, I noticed something incredible- I actually felt GOOD. The whole thing just seemed so funny and ridiculous to me that the nerves fled my body and allowed me to continue approaching other girls who caught my eye.

I'd also keep approaching until I could finally end on a high note. Somehow at the time, I intuitively understood the conditioning principle. If I went home after a bad rejection, it'd make me not want to go back out the next night. Instead, I'd tell myself after every rejection, "one last approach." This became a mantra for me, and I'd do approach after approach (all of which were rejections) until I finally hit it off with one girl, or maybe even got a number. While you'll soon learn the various skills that go with approaching a girl correctly at the end of the day, it's also just a numbers game. The more you approach, the better chance you have of one going well. As Wayne Gretzky once put it, "You miss 100% of the shots that you don't take."

I mentioned earlier about having a mantra, but the truth is I used several to help keep my head in the game. Whether it was "be comfortable being uncomfortable," "it's just practice," or the very crude "fuck it" before immediately approaching, each mantra and mentality helped give me that extra push. Often when working with a student, I'll help them develop their own personal mantra. Something they can say over and over again that makes them more comfortable and even gives them a feeling of power when out and approaching. One student will always say "I'm home" when he walks into a bar, which instantly relaxes him; another student uses an amusing "Unleash the beast" to give him a sense of power. There really isn't any wrong mantra per se. The key is that whatever mantra you use does two incredibly important things.

First, your mantra should hammer in a key point. If I say to myself when out, "How do I want to remember this moment?", it reminds me that in a few hours all of this will just be a memory. It's up to me whether I want this memory to be a good one or a bad one. All I need to do is take the actions I know, in this case approaching when I see a girl I like, and even if it doesn't go well, I can be proud of myself for the action taken. Remember the importance identity plays in all this?

Second, your mantra should make you FEEL something. Maybe it's happy, or a sense of confidence. Whatever it may be, a mantra isn't effective unless you get a small positive feeling shooting through your body. Typically shorter and more crude mantras do the trick. It's your mantra, remember, so no need to be poetic. It just needs to get the job done, by giving you a small emotional boost.

These positive boosts can come from the most unlikely, and sometimes quite ridiculous, places. When I first started approaching, I would hum the Mario theme song in my head, as I walked around looking for girls. Sure, it's silly, but it did something very important; it gave me a constant reminder that this was no different than playing a video game.

People can use multiple concepts to frame what they're doing. One frame/perspective is that I'm putting my self worth on the line and allowing myself to be judged by each girl I come across. *Ouch.* That hurts even thinking about it. Another frame, though, is that this is a make believe world that has no real negative consequences on my life. Sounds a lot better, doesn't it?

I've played with a ton of these different frames and used a few analogies to make sure I'm thinking about this the right way. One analogy is that I'm plugged into the Matrix, and every thing and every person around me is just code in a program. If you're a sci-fi nerd like me, then you might like to pretend it's the holo-deck on Star Trek. Perhaps you're just seeing it as a video game, where every rejection just means you can respawn at the last checkpoint and try again. Hopefully you see what these all have in common: it's not the "real world."

When we look at the "real world," we automatically assume that it's anything we come into contact with or anything our senses experience. But to help overcome my own approach and social anxiety, I give it a completely different meaning. I see the real world as anything that has *significance* to my life. Sure, there's somewhere in Denmark right now where there's a gorgeous girl, but I'll never meet her so, what do I care what she thinks? Unless something adds significance to my life, I treat it as simply a playground or video game. This leads to another mantra of mine, and probably the most important: "It's no big deal."

If you can internalize that philosophy, that most things in life aren't a big deal, you'll be miles ahead of everyone else trying to master the art of the approach. Try the following exercise.

Go out until you see a girl you find attractive and approach her if you can, though if you can't, that's fine too. Either way, rate on a scale of 1-10 how big a deal it felt to go talk to her before you made the attempt. Then the next day, think back, and again rate on a scale of 1-10 how big a deal you think it was. Pretty crazy, huh?

In the moment, our brain plays tricks on us and floods us with panic. Don't be too angry with it though, it's actually trying to help you. Due to all the reasons I mentioned in the previous chapter, your brain will do anything it can to stop you from approaching when you want to. For beginners, it's pure panic. For intermediate guys, it's faulty logic; they might think, for example, that it can't work because of some random factor, so why bother? For advanced guys, it's ego based, where they don't want to risk seeing a negative reaction that challenges their ego.

If we can push past the excuses our brains give us though, then it reverses and takes away the anxiety, or at least lessens it. Most guys who've tried a few approaches know exactly what I'm talking about. You see the girl and feel the panic, yet force yourself to just put one foot in front of the other and walk up to her anyway. The moment you finally open your mouth and she responds, though, you realize that feeling has dissipated. This may not be true for everyone, since some guys struggle deeply on keeping a conversation going and run into those incredibly awkward pauses. Once that skill set is learned, though, everyone realizes the quickest way to get rid of the approach anxiety is to approach. It's an instant relief.

Let's take this time and go over some tips and tricks you can do right there on the spot, to help make the approach happen in the first place. One thing is to treat it like a band-aid. The longer you stand around thinking about approaching, you're just giving your anxiety time to build. You'll never push the anxiety down, you just need to get it over with as quickly as possible. To do this, try seeing the girl you like and then saying, "1, 2, 3...Go!" No matter what, once you say go, you need to walk over to her and begin talking.

Congrats! You bit the bullet and did your first approach of the night. Remember what I said earlier, though? We need back-to-back approaches to build momentum and get you in a good state, where it stops being so scary. A fun way to do this is by giving yourself a countdown. Once I finish talking to a girl, I'll immediately begin counting down from 30 out loud. "30...29...28...27," and no matter what, I refuse to get to 1 before I'm talking to the next girl. If you can do this five times, you'll quickly start noticing that "no big deal" philosophy begin to take hold.

Other guys I've encountered, though, would rather just get over it in one big go. This is similar to doing a cannonball in the deep end of the pool versus going in bit by bit. If you feel you're more in this category, there's a few fun things you can do that will almost instantly snap you into the right headspace. It may take more than one try, but it's definitely faster than anything else.

The secret? Go get rejected on *purpose*.

There's three main ways to go about doing this. The first way entails finding the bitchiest, hottest, and just flat out most intimidating girl you can find. When you see her, you say the scariest and most raw thing you can imagine. For me, it's usually something very direct. For example, "You are the most gorgeous girl in here, and I'm incredibly attracted to you. I have to meet you." If she responds positively, then you just hit the jackpot! More likely she'll give an awkward laugh and thank you, but then excuse herself in some way. It's honestly unimportant. What you'll realize after this, is that you just did the hardest approach possible and lived to tell the tale. Anything, now, compared to that, will seem like a cakewalk.

Another way is to tap into your silly side. Self-amusement is damn near critical if you're going to survive learning this skill. To do this, just start approaching in ways that will make you laugh and put no importance on how the girl responds. Often, my friends and I will challenge each other with silly openers. They can range from asking the girl if she's accepted Jesus Christ as her lord and savior, to hopping on one foot the entire time. What's important is that YOU think it's funny and will get a laugh out of it. By treating it as a fun and silly game that doesn't matter, it becomes a fun and silly game that doesn't matter. Shocker, I know.

Finally, you can just say screw it and flat out ask to get rejected. What's really funny about this approach is not only does it help get rid of the anxiety, but a good amount of the time she'll laugh and continue talking with you. Think about it: what guy says that to a girl? I'm not saying this is by any means the most effective approach, but for just a way to get out of your head, it's not half bad.

In my years of coaching, I've seen some of the most extreme examples of approach anxiety, and in some cases, you just need real consequences if YOU don't approach. One student I had years ago, Dan, just wouldn't approach, no matter how much I encouraged him. Finally, I had enough and told him to give me his car keys. When he did, I explained he's not driving home until he's approached 10 different women. If I had to wait there until morning, so be it. He begged, he bargained, he even threatened to physically try and take them from me. In the end, though, he did the approaches and thanked me, since he finally broke through the fear.

You may not need to go to these extremes yourself, but having a buddy to hold you accountable can do wonders. By using the commitment principle to your advantage, overcoming the approach anxiety can become possible. There's different ways to use it, and I recommend trying them all out to see which works strongest for you.

One way is to tell your friends that you're going to approach a certain number of girls tonight, no matter what. With the expectations on you, it becomes much harder to punk out. My friend and prominent dating coach, DJ Fuji, would often tap a random guy on the shoulder, telling him to call him a bitch if he didn't talk to a certain girl. Once the guy said it, he'd be too ashamed not to approach.

Of course, you can always put money on it, as well. Loads of my students will give each other $200, or an amount that's enough incentive for him, and, after every approach, have that friend give him $20 back. By giving yourself some consequences, whether it's emotional or physical, you'll have a much better shot at reaching your goals for the night.

In summary, the main objective here is to get momentum going, in any way possible. Remember, every action you take either leads to more or less anxiety. The quicker you get approaching, the quicker you can overcome it. I urge you to constantly view this process using the correct frames I suggested above, and actively practice the tips for when you're out.

With all that said, a lot of the work to not only get over the fear of approaching, but to make it work at all, starts before you even leave the house. I'm now going to show you all the little things guys do wrong, before they even see a girl they like. Use it correctly and you'll have an unbeatable edge on every other guy out there.

Ch. 3 Prerequisites To The Approach

It always astounds me how people still, with everything we know, just want a quick fix. We know fully well that anything worth having requires hard work. We know that every successful and extraordinary human being didn't get that way with, "just one simple trick." Yet even with unlimited examples of greatness telling the world what it takes, the vast majority of people look for the easiest solution. *Don't be the vast majority of people.*

To become successful at approaching means putting in the work, *before you ever approach.* This includes:

1. Fashion
2. Grooming

3. Preparing yourself and place

4. Learning body language

5. Having a plan

6. Warming up

7. Memorizing and practicing openers

Every single workshop I do begins the exact same way. Everyone sits down, eager to hear a long speech and take notes, but quickly realizes that, one by one, they will need to explain why they wore whatever it is they wore. Maybe their jeans are 10 years old or look like they belong to a painter. Perhaps their shirt is two sizes too big. On one occasion, I had a 72 year old man show up wearing a T-shirt with a bedazzled skull on the center, a leather fedora hat, a rocker style spiked bracelet, cargo shorts, and sandals. Now I know what you may be thinking. You like your clothes and they fit all right; no they don't. The vast majority of men have no idea how to dress, or at least in a way that's attractive to girls.

While what you wear does matter, the most important thing for any style you choose is the fit. I'd suggest getting three really money outfits, ones you'd see a celebrity wear, that probably would make you a little uncomfortable. When you have them, get them tailored. You probably spent hundreds on them, if done right, so why not spend a little more so that they actually work? Don't cheap out on this.

To figure out an attractive style that works for you, start a look book. Go online and look up celebrities and models who have roughly the same type of face and build you have. If you're over or under weight, just pick the closest match you can. With that said though, getting in better shape not only makes any outfit look ten times better, but also greatly improves your chances of a successful approach.

Once you have your look book, go out to the mall. I do mean the mall by the way. Remember the importance of a good fit? Once you're at the mall, begin trying to replicate the outfits in your look book as best you can.

Pro tip 1: Approach and ask women for their opinions on items you're deciding on. You'll be surprised at how helpful they can be and you just might hit it off, too.

Pro tip 2: Go on-line and look up donsfootwear.com. They have great looking shoes that will discreetly give you 2-4 inches of extra height. I've never had a girl call me out or care if I told her, either.

Pro tip 3: Wear something outside your comfort zone. Maybe it's a funny shirt, a cool bracelet or necklace, or an edgy hairstyle. It's important to stand out from the crowd and have a conversation piece on you, as well.

Fashion is, by far, the easiest thing to fix and, after just one trip to the mall, it can drastically improve your chances of a girl being receptive towards you. Equally as easy to do and just as important is a man's grooming, as well. It's always uncomfortable and a bit embarrassing, but every now and then, I'll need to take one of my students aside to tell him he smells. This can be from lack of showering or using deodorant, but either way, I send him home to fix it before we continue.

If it's not yet obvious to you, shower regularly, put on deodorant every morning, brush your teeth, and don't wear a pound of cologne. No matter how skilled you get talking to girls, you have to realize that if you smell in any way, that's a deal breaker. You literally become unbearable to be around, not to mention all the subtle signals you're sending about how you don't respect yourself.

Beyond smell, grooming includes paying attention to the little things, because believe me, women notice everything. When I go and get my haircut, I make sure it's a full service salon. This means I can have my ears and nose waxed, my eyebrows done to prevent uni-brow, and beard perfectly trimmed and lined up neatly. It's a little extra money, sure, but do you really want your dream girl focusing on that one stray nose hair while you're talking to her?

Keep in mind this doesn't mean becoming a full metro-sexual and obsessing about your looks. Tons of women have told me consistently that they don't want a guy who's prettier than them or looks like he takes two hours getting ready. It just means you should look *clean.* So while you don't need to be getting weekly manicures, you should notice if you have any obvious dirt under your nails.

I sincerely hope, before moving on, that you take the time to go out and get some proper outfits and make sure you're clean. Remember, any time you leave the house, you should be looking your best, because you never know if that's the day you meet an attractive girl. Fate usually has a sadistic sense of humor and will punish you by doing just that.

Before going out, even if you're looking your best, you now need to begin doing some prep work. What this means, in the big scope of things, is plan on succeeding. Most guys go out and have the limiting belief that, even if they meet a girl, it's just a fantasy that she'll be into him. This messes them up, not only psychologically, but logistically as well. Always plan for success.

What does successful planning look like? For starters, it means carrying a condom on you whenever you leave the house. I'm not going to spend time here going over the importance of safe sex; just don't be an idiot. It's obviously good to have when needed, and there's a psychological boost that comes from carrying it around, just knowing sex is on the table.

One of my best friends and wingman is obsessed with good breath, too. Not only will he always make sure to be carrying around mints and mouth spray, but he stores mouthwash in his car's glove compartment, "just in case." Is it a bit much? Sure, but you'll never see him getting rejected due to his smell, either.

Preparing yourself is only half of it though, because there's a much bigger issue: your place. You have to assume that when out meeting women, and people in general, someone may be coming back to your place. It could be just a romantic/sexual encounter with a girl you met, or it can be a group of 20 rowdy new friends you just made. Whatever the case may be, nothing brings down the vibe like not having your place in order.

Having your place clean goes without saying. It can still look lived in, but there shouldn't be a mountain of clothes on the floor or dishes in the sink. This all comes back again to what I said about displaying your respect and care about yourself. Your environment reflects what kind of man you are, so treat it right.

Besides just the cleanliness, there's the ambiance to think of, as well. Invest in some form of sound system, and have the best of different music genres ready to be played. You never know if your guest(s) prefer rap, top 40, or EDM, so be prepared for it all. Lighting also does wonders, as well, to keep the party vibe going. Most likely you were just in a dark club or bar; coming back to bright lights everywhere can be a massive state break.

To combat this, you should invest in either dimming lights or LED light-bulbs that change color. My neighbor and friend pimped out his place with LED lights all along the wall that will actually flash and change color with the music that's being played. It's very entertaining and keeps everyone in a fun mood. None of this matters, though, without the ultimate preparation for a fun mood: alcohol.

If your place isn't stocked with liquor, don't even bother bringing people over. Everything quickly becomes awkward, and you'll ruin the great thing you just built all night. If you don't know much about the different liquor types and mixers, take the time and do a simple google search. You don't need to become an expert, by any means, but you should at least know the basics.

On average, your safest bet is always Vodka. You can mix this with cranberry, orange juice, Sprite...practically anything really. Having whiskey and coke, or shots of tequila hanging around, doesn't hurt either. While most people aren't too picky, there are some who are very particular, so the more variety the better. The best part is, liquor takes forever to go bad, unlike beer, so it should last you a good while.

Next up, we need to do something about the way you carry yourself. The average man has terrible posture from either slouching or just looking closed off. I could write an entire book on just body language, but there's already a million out there. Stop what you're doing right now and buy one. I guarantee you don't know nearly as much as you think you do.

I have two basic rules I tell all my students regarding body language:

1. Be as comfortable or more comfortable than the girl
2. Be as invested or less invested than the girl

To start off, find your neutral position. It's surprisingly very easy. Simply put your back against the wall and make sure every part of you touches the wall, including your head and heels. Don't worry if part of your back is arched and doesn't touch; just do the best you can. Now step forward holding that exact same position. The result should be good posture. You can also always imagine a string pulling the top of your head up and a rod going down your back, but my way just seems less painful.

While you're out, you want to do everything you can to appear confident and comfortable. This means no crossing your arms, hands in pockets, high shoulders, darting eye movement, and so on. Again, I really recommend you buy a comprehensive body language book so you can eliminate all the signs that even hint at nervousness. It's instant value for your dollar, and you'll be using that knowledge for every encounter you have.

What you won't find is proper body language during an approach, so that's what I'd like to focus on here. If you've ever seen a guy approach a girl in the bar, it's usually one of three ways. The first has him going directly up to her as she's leaning on the bar, and facing her directly, as he uses his line. In this case, he's breaking both of my rules: he's way more invested and he's clearly less comfortable. Sadly this is the typical approach I see.

Some guys with "game" try the other two methods. The second is where the guy walks up and leans up against the bar himself, before facing the girl and trying out his opener. Think of the typical player scenario where a guy has his arm up against the wall and is extra close to the girl. This guy is as comfortable, but he's still more invested.

Finally, we have the third approach that only became popular from men trying to learn this. They'll typically walk next to the girl, but then turn their backs to them and try opening over their shoulder. It looks as silly as it reads. In this approach they're trying not to show any interest, but by doing so, make the whole interaction seem awkward or off-putting. They're less invested in the girl, but they substituted being as comfortable.

What I like to do is approach as if you are walking by and happened to notice her. Your body language shouldn't indicate you're there to pick her up, unless you did a direct approach, but we'll get into that later. Instead, you want to give off that she just happened to be in your area and something caught your attention about her. To do this right, you should, as quickly as possible, be mirroring the way she's facing and also lean on anything in proximity. This will all make more sense after you do a few approaches, but just remember to keep an eye out for how you can invest less with your body while also becoming more comfortable.

Before we move on, I do want to point out that sometimes there's just no way to do the above. Maybe she's sitting down and there's no chair, so you're forced to stand. In this case, you can't be as comfortable as her. Does that mean you shouldn't approach? Of course not. It just means, do the best you can. I've often approached and, if the girl's receptive, walked a bit away to find another chair, and brought it back. Doesn't that make the interaction a little awkward? Absolutely, but I'd rather have a few seconds of awkwardness over a slow gradual weirdness, that creeps in from standing the entire time while she's sitting.

The last thing I want to address about body language and mannerisms is the importance of animation. Every single bootcamp I run, and I mean EVERY, we address this problem. Guys are just conditioned since birth not to emote, and instead play it very chill and suave. This works wonders in movies but doesn't do anything for you in the real world, *unless the girl is already attracted to you.* Instead, we need to rely on animation. Women are emotional creatures, and will have greater emotional responses to what you say, and be a million times more engaged with you, if you're lively.

I want to be clear, though, that being animated doesn't mean be loud and have wild movements. Every single one of my students makes this mistake at first. What good animation means is basically good acting, using hand gestures and facial expressions to really convey the emotion of everything you're saying. If you've ever seen "Ferris Bueller's Day Off," think of his teacher calling his name. That's a prime example for lack of animation. If you've ever seen almost any Ryan Reynolds movie, ever, especially Van Wilder, you'll see what I mean when talking about good animation.

After you've learned the core concepts of good body language, it's time to start taking action. Does that mean approaching every girl in sight? Does it mean going over your schedule to figure out what nights you'll go out? It could. It's really up to you. To do this properly, though, you need to make a plan of action on how you're going to learn this. I promise if you just wing it and hope for the best, you will 100% fail.

Unfortunately I don't know your schedule, what you do, or the time constraints you have. I can give you what I did when I first started, and what I generally require from my students. When I began approaching I was obsessed; you couldn't keep me in the house. I'd be going out six nights a week, and would average around 20 approaches, because they went by so fast. Thankfully, you don't need to do all that to improve your skill. It just shows you that, like anything else in the world, good things come to those who work hard.

Typically my students are required to do three essential things when going out. First, they need to commit to going out 2-4 times a week. I think four is the magic number but, at the very least, commit to two. Second, they need to commit to the number of girls that they'll be approaching when out. It's very easy to go out and approach, "here and there" but that always leads to inaction and not getting much done. Force yourself to get 10 approaches each night you go out, and find a way to keep yourself accountable. The third thing, a real key rule, and that's to approach the first girl you see when walking into the venue.

Remember how I said that anxiety is a spectrum, and it's either getting worse or getting better? This makes use of that rule immediately. Most guys will walk in and check their phones, or go to the bathroom, or get a drink, or a million other things to waste time. All this does is give your anxiety a chance to grow! Instead, by approaching the first girl you see, you'll instantly shock your system and get off on the right foot. Every approach after that will start to get easier, and you'll learn a golden rule: *if you start the night strong, you'll finish strong*

By having these set rules and plans of action in place, you're setting yourself up for success. The approach of the first girl you see, and preferably quick approach of any other girl you see, also serves another purpose. That purpose is simply warming up. Ideally, if you go to the gym, you'll stretch first, or do some light weights to warm up. Pitchers, before going on the plate, will toss the ball a few times before warming up, as well. Getting the night going to have successful approaches is no different. You must have a warm up phase.

Here's a common scenario: a guy works long hours at his job where he's stuck in his head all day. If he has any social interactions, they're very limited and always professional. He's tired, stressed, and just doesn't have a lot of energy. This man comes home and eats a meal watching TV, still in his head, and realizes he's supposed to go out tonight to work on his approach. He changes his clothes and gets ready, then drives in silence, at best with the radio on, before parking and walking up to the bar. After all this, once he walks inside, he realizes he needs to now have the gift of gab, act super animated, and be approaching everyone in sight. He then proceeds to shit himself, and become a wall flower for the rest of the night.

Moral of the story, don't be this guy. I understand you're busy; we all are. I also understand that you work long hours, are usually in your head, and just want the nights or weekends to relax. All I can say is, *suck it the fuck up*. If this were easy, everyone would be doing it, and it wouldn't be worth having.

The good news is that by going through a steady warm up structure before you ever leave the house, you can help negate all these problems.

Most men will just use booze as a way to get out of their heads. This is terrible for building your core confidence and ability to learn and retain information. Do this sober or, if it's truly unbearable, allow yourself only one shot before leaving the house. No buying drinks when out. Instead, we're going to rely on self-amusement and techniques that turn our internal focus into external focus.

After I finish my day and realize it's time to go out, the very first thing I do is blast music in my room. Play music that you want to sing along to or dance to or anything that generally pumps you up into a good mood. Get in the shower, and start singing a song. From here on out you should be speaking as much as possible. This starts telling your brain to get used to speaking instead of just thinking everything.

When getting ready in front of the mirror, try saying fun

positive affirmations. It may sound a bit douchey, but I'll

usually just mention words of encouragement like, "Damn,

look at this sexy guy, you're going to kill it tonight." Make sure

you put on your favorite outfit. Something you feel money in.

Often just the way you dress and groom and put detail into

your look also gets your mood and confidence up as well.

Again, throughout this whole process, I'm just talking to myself

or, if I have a friend with me, engaging in constant chatter.

On the way to the venue, I'll once again play my favorite

songs. Unlike the previous guy though, I'll be singing at the

top of my lungs, smiling and nodding to other cars who pull up

beside me, and self-amuse myself with any funny

observations I make about the things I see during the ride

there.

After I pull up and park and get in line, small talk will usually

occur with whoever's around me. Simple compliments and

greetings, nothing high pressure or long needed conversation.

I'm simply keeping my mouth working. Ideally, I'll also talk with the bouncer or anyone who works there. This is especially important for social life hacks if you continue to go to the same bar or place.

Now that I'm finally inside, the last phase of my warm up begins: approaching! The first group I see, I'm in and fully ready to crash and burn; I may even open with something silly, just to amuse myself. Usually the first 10 minutes of the night doesn't matter anyway.

Hopefully from reading the two scenarios above, you can easily see what a drastic difference there will be between the first and second guy, once he first makes it into the bar. Don't ignore these steps because again, if you start strong, you'll finish strong. No one, not even myself, is above the fundamentals, and if something works, you should always use it to ensure a good night.

With all this said, it's time to talk about the key reason I'm sure everyone bought this book in the first place. Which is: getting into the nitty gritty of what to say and having some great lines you can use immediately tonight. I do want to stress that eventually, you'll want to be able to generate openers on the spot from something situational (more on this in the next chapter) but it's always good to have something to fall back on.

Any night you're out, have at least three openers prepared that you've actually practiced multiple times in front of the mirror. This doesn't just mean remember the words, but the proper delivery, as well. Does your facial expressions make sense? Is your tonality conveying the right emotion? What does your body language communicate as you're saying this? You need to answer all the questions to pull off any of these openers. So try them out, and drill them in front of the mirror first. Then when you're ready, let's go get your first approaches in.

Ch. 4 Openers

What's funny about approaching women, and the openers you use in general, is that it's both the least important and most important step in building attraction. This is because once you're comfortable with opening, you'll quickly realize almost anything works. As I've stated before, I've probably done 10,000 or more approaches, and I doubt any one of the women truly remembers how the conversation started. The vibe and flow of conversation following the opener matters, of course, and will lead to the girl either being receptive or closed off; but not so much the initial opener.

On the other hand, it's important, because nothing else can happen without taking this crucial step. Not only that, but first impressions matter, and how you decide to open will dictate the flow, in some part, of the interaction. She has no idea who you are, what your intentions are, or even if you're a threat or not. This is why putting your best foot forward from the beginning can give you crucial time to make the impression you desire.

As for the openers themselves, I'd like you to imagine them within a spectrum that leads from an indirect style of approach to a direct style of approach. Everyone reading this is different, and based on looks, predispositions, comfort, and of course, trial and error, will be able to choose which style(s) works best for him.

Indirect   Direct

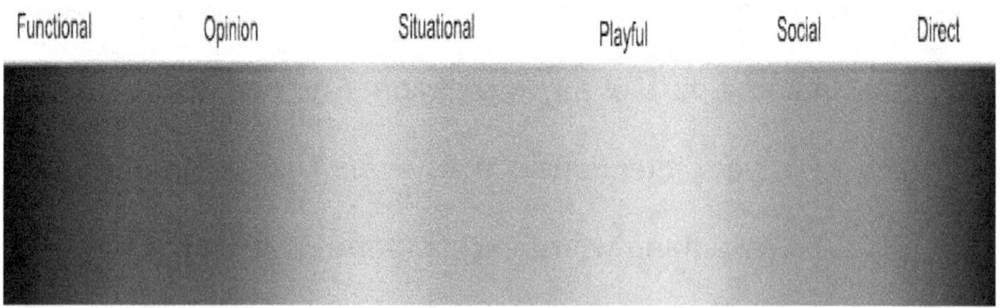

Functional:

The most indirect style, by far, is what we call the functional opener. It's anything you can ask someone that is completely within the social norms, things people will often ask strangers when it's a necessity. Delivery is meant to be acted out as if you sincerely needed to know what you're asking and give off the illusion that the only reason you asked the girl was because she just happened to be in your proximity.

Strengths:

This can usually open about anything unless someone is *really* having a bad day. It's great for those with crippling anxiety, because there's no real way you can get rejected from this alone. For those who are new, it can usually be a good way to begin the warm up portion of the night, as well. If you've used a functional opener and had a positive demeanor the entire time, it's perfectly fine to approach the same girl again a little bit later; it can even help!

Weakness:

This opener is notoriously difficult to turn into actual back and forth conversation. Don't get me wrong, there are ways, but it takes a great deal of acting and the ability to think on your feet. For example, if, after I used my functional opener, I just happened to notice she has a slight accent, I can become curious where she's from, and how I'm jealous I don't have a cool British accent.

Functional Examples:

1. Excuse me, but would you happen to know where the nearest coffee shop is?
2. I'm sorry but I think my phone is off. Can you tell me what time it is?

3. Would you happen to know where the bathroom is, by any chance?

4. Excuse me, I have some friends meeting me here from X bar. Do you know how far that is from here?

5. Hey there, you wouldn't happen to know when the main DJ comes on, would you?

Opinion:

For the longest time, this was easily the bread and butter for anyone learning how to attract women. The concept is quite simple: you're walking by and, after noticing the girl, would like a random person's opinion on something. I'll often go a step further and get into a fake argument with my friend loud enough for them to hear before approaching. This style of opening is solely meant to convey that you would just like her thoughts; nothing about it should indicate you're interested in the girl or trying to hit on her. Of course, just the act of any guy coming up and making conversation has a girl suspecting your intentions, but it leaves nothing for her to directly call out.

Strengths:

The opener itself has built-in conversation topics that you can discuss with the girl you like and her friends. Everyone likes to have her opinions valued as well, so it also plays upon her vanity. If done right, you can get approaches in that may seem awkward or uncomfortable for the girl if obvious intentions were known. I also prefer this style for more low energy environments, such as a girl quietly eating her dinner in a restaurant.

Weakness:

It's extremely easy to get lost in the initial topic that the opinion is about. While not as hard to transition out of a functional opener, it can still be challenging for newer guys. Once you've spent a few minutes going back and forth on what everyone thinks, it becomes awkward to suddenly change gears into something different. There's also no underlying flirtatiousness, which absolutely doesn't need to be the case when opening, but it does mean that it becomes easier to get stuck in purely platonic conversation.

Opinion Opener Examples:

1. Hey, I need a random person's opinion on something. My niece just turned 18 last week, and she wants to get a tattoo, but I don't think she should. Is it my place to say something? (they answer) Sure, but here's the thing...she wants a tattoo of her current boyfriend's name. What are your thoughts now?

2. Hey guys, I could use a ladies insight on this. My buddy has been on a bunch of dates with this girl he really likes, but she never pays for anything, doesn't even offer. At one point does a guy need to stop paying for every date, and how do you go about that conversation?

3. Excuse me, maybe you can settle a debate between me and my friend here. He says straight men can't be into romantic comedies without a girl thinking he's instantly gay. Is that true?

4. [For hard to reach groups, usually sitting off by themselves or in a booth] Hey guys, I have a random question for you and hope you can help me out. My buddy and I were talking about how no one meets in person anymore, but mainly online now. If a guy was to try and meet you in person, how could he go about it with all of you over here? What would be a smooth way?

5. Hey guys, maybe you can help me out with something. My friend Karen has been dating this guy Mark for a few months now. Recently she went to a party, got drunk, and made out with a girl there. He says that's cheating and is really upset, but she doesn't consider that actually cheating. Who's right here, and what should he do?

Situational:

If you've ever seen a really smooth and natural approach in a movie or TV show, chances are they used a situational approach. It's the ideal "natural" way to meet someone, especially in the girls' mind. Usually a situation presents itself and the guy, seeing his window of opportunity, does or mentions something based on what he saw. It should be slightly out of the ordinary. Try and see what sticks out. In the movie "Hitch," we see a funny fabricated situational opener. The guy is lying on the street, holding the girls puppy who ran away, and is just short of a car that supposedly almost ran him over. Men will go to great lengths to make it seem that the initial meeting "just happened" through no fault of their own. If done properly, it will leave the girl guessing, "Did he want to come talk to me or did the situation just warrant it?"

Strengths:

This is by far the most preferred approach by advanced guys. If done right, it makes the approach extremely comfortable for the girl, because it's low investment and has a built in talking topic. Often it doesn't even seem like an approach at all; instead it's as if you were striking up a conversation with a friend. This style can be used anywhere, and gives major points for seeming non-needy and being socially intelligent.

Weakness:

It's preferred by advanced guys because it's a very advanced form of opening. For starters, you need to be able to see a good situational reason to start a conversation. This isn't always available. What's worse, when guys try and force it by mentioning something obvious or random, it can lead to a very awkward interaction. Not that we should care, it's all practice after all, but it can be pretty tricky to pull off. It can also be abrupt and awkward if there's not a good transition or follow-up. The idea is you started talking about the situation, and switched gears to ask her name or where she's from, and ruined that effect.

Situational Opener Examples:

1. (Spots girl dancing drunkenly on the bar) Bartender said you're next...hope you got some moves.

2. (Noticing the girls are wearing near identical outfits) OK, who copied who here?

3. (Girl is wearing very high uncomfortable looking shoes) Hey, on a scale of 1-10, how bad do your feet hurt right now?

4. (Girl is looking at a menu) Ooooh, you don't want to get that one.

5. (Group of girls are staring intensely at a crowd) Wow, this is some extreme people watching, huh?

Playful:

At this point we're going more towards the direct end of the spectrum. Playful and onwards is seen as direct simply because you're owning the fact that you wanted to come talk to her. Personally I love the playful style the best, with situational being a strong number two; to each his own, though. The idea of the playful opener is to get a laugh and set a good mood right from the start. Yes, you came over just to talk to her, but it should be more about having a fun time and self-amusement than anything else. Chances are, if you don't find the opener fun and playful, she won't either, so make sure it's something that gets a smile from you first.

Strengths:

If you can keep a girl smiling and laughing, she's yours. This style is a great way to show the fun side of your personality and is a breath of fresh air from the boring style most men use. It allows for a battle of wits, which can make transitioning into normal, or fun, conversation much easier. If done well, you'll notice the girls being much more receptive and welcoming than normal.

Weakness:

Unfortunately a playful style isn't for everyone. Some men have a hard time projecting it correctly, and when they try, it looks forced and uncomfortable. Some women also may find it weird or not know how to respond. Unfortunately it's hard to know before the approach, so can be hit or miss at times. Finally, because it's on the direct end of the spectrum, the girls may not want to play along, because they can tell you're trying to hit on them.

Playful Opener Examples:

1. Oh my god, I was going to wear the exact same outfit tonight. How embarrassing would that be? (she answers) To be fair, I do have the ass for it.

2. Hey, I'm so sorry, but we received multiple noise complaints about you guys. I'm going to have to ask you keep it down. Sorry, I don't make the rules.

3. Wow, I am so sorry I'm late for our date; traffic was rough. You brought your friends along I see.

4. Hey, I saw you staring at my chest and I'm very flattered. (She denies it) Oh, of course not; I wouldn't

admit it either, if it was me. Just remember, I'm not just

a piece of meat, though, and we'll be fine.

5. Hey, can you take a heartfelt, sincere compliment from

    someone? (she responds) OK, well I can for sure.

    Here, you go first.

Social:

Social direct is best used for new guys attempting this. The

reason is because any opener really works; they're not meant

to be magic lines that make attraction instant. By using social

openers, you realize you can talk with anyone and don't need

a gimmick. While it's true some openers are best for certain

situations, most guys forget how a simple hello can do. The

idea of social openers is to simply own the fact that you want

to talk to them. If done right, you should come across as a

very confident and friendly guy.

Strengths:

The strength here is confidence. Most guys always need something witty to say. By going direct, you're showing you don't need to hide behind any "lines." Unlike situational, the social openers practically work everywhere. This instantly takes away the excuse of, "I don't know what to say." When in doubt, just go with a social opener.

Weakness:

While it does give points for confidence, it also clearly shows your intention of wanting to meet, and most likely, pick up the girl. If the girl isn't in a receptive mood, doesn't like your look, or just in a high energy state, this style of approach may feel like going uphill. It also doesn't allow for much built in conversation topics; this means transitioning from the opener can be tough, as well.

Social Opener Examples:

1. Hey, you guys seem fun; just wanted to come by and say hi.

2. Hey there, I don't believe I've met you yet.

3. (Raise a glass to clink hers) Cheers!

4. (Friend introduces you even though he doesn't know her)

5. Hey, what's your name?

Direct:

It should be understood that some differentiate direct from sexual direct. As for me, I see both having the same effect; one is just more shocking than the other. Direct boils down to showing absolute confidence in your desire and not wasting any time. While this is always OK to do as a man, it should be understood that "going direct" isn't an excuse to sexually harass or cat call to a girl. That style never works and can get you into some trouble. Instead, it's all about cutting to the chase in a way she can respect.

Strengths:

If a girl is receptive off a direct approach, half the job is done. There's very little in terms of playing games. If done well, a direct approach can also be highly arousing to the girl. Surprisingly, this approach does the best in environments with no alcohol. This is because she knows it's truly you and not just liquid courage.

Weakness:

This is by far the most typical style girls get from drunk guys at the bar. Because of this, you can be perceived the same way, which makes you look desperate and needy. Often this style works if the girl already is thinking of you in a non-platonic way; for example, she's noticed you in a high status role or likes the way you look. It is true that direct is preferred for the daytime, or places with no alcohol. But in bars and nightclubs, it rarely works out well.

Direct Opener Examples:

1. I'm sorry, but if I didn't come over and say hi I'd be kicking myself in the ass all day.

2. Wow, you are so incredibly sexy.

3. Hey, I saw you over there and thought you're absolutely gorgeous, so I needed to come say hi.

4. I never do this, but something about you made me need to come over and see what you're about.

5. I just have to say you look stunning. I saw you and knew I had to come meet you.

Whatever opener you prefer, I suggest trying them all, multiple times. It's good not to rely too heavily on any one thing. If a certain opener scares you more than another, then you should definitely practice that one, as well. Remember, a large part of this is developing your core confidence. If you rely too heavily on the lines and forget the fundamentals needed, then none of these approaches will work for you. This is why I waited towards near the end to share them with you. I wanted you to see that so much, such as fashion, body language, your mental state, the way you approach, the situation, and your personal style all come into play.

Epilogue: Moving Forward

As I've mentioned before, approaching is just the start, literally. It's not meant to get her to want to date you. Any girl that would after any line would be a complete nut job. Instead, you're to use the tools provided here to help get you out there and meeting as many as possible.

By realizing rejection is part of the dating game, you can constantly refine and perfect your approach. This is only the beginning though, because there are hundreds of social skills you can develop that will not only help your dating goals, but make life itself better. I have had students all over the world use techniques I've taught them to not just have sexual adventures, but also to get married, get promotions, grow a social circle, and have insane connections. The sky's the limit, really, when you know how to interact with people well.

To give you an example, here are just some of the most basic things you can develop, things I help my students grow every day:

- Sexually escalating
- Managing relationships
- Not running out of things
- Body language and tonality
- Being funny
- Being dominant
- Controlling people's perceptions
- Making plans with people that don't flake

The list goes on and on really. If you're serious about this aspect of your life, then you need to put in the time and effort to make a permanent change. We see it all the time with health and wealth. Guys will spend hours in the gym and do strict meal prep to get the body they want. We also see guys working long hours and grinding away to better their life financially. So why should this be any different?

For those who are ready to reach their true potential, I'll let you know the formula that every successful person has used:

First thing is you need to practice. I mean, be almost obsessed with it. When I first started learning this, you couldn't keep me in the house. I was out at least six nights a week, approaching everyone in sight. Whether it was trying to get a date or just make a friend, I knew it required relentless repetition. That's not to say that you need to go as extreme as I did, but you should understand that more is always better. I suggest 3-4 times a week for going out and practicing. Basically use the same rule you'd use for going to the gym. I doubt there's a single guy with your ideal body who goes to the gym only once a week.

The second thing is you need to play smart. Take notes and organize them. Don't flood yourself with information; instead, learn only what you need for the next step to succeed. Once you're able to do that, then move on to other stuff. This book is an excellent start for the basics and gives you more than enough to practice, for now. Realize it's not meant to be grueling work; you should be able to find the fun in the process, to avoid getting burned out. I'd also keep track of how each night goes, so you can analyze what to do differently next time.

Finally, you need a mentor. You can't know the right way to go by searching blind, or if you do, it'll take a decade. Having someone better than you, even slightly, can help you develop the tools you need to succeed. For those who want even more benefits, a good mentor will also keep you accountable. It's easy to start slacking when it's just yourself; The main reason why people have personal trainers is just to ensure they show up to the gym. Also keep in mind, choosing the right mentor is tricky, and choosing the wrong mentor can be a waste of time, or even install bad habits. I can't tell you how many dating coaches I've seen who would get drunk on the job, steal a girl from his client, not pay attention to him, or just give him flat out awful advice.

For those who are serious, who want someone personally looking out for their success, then I'm always available. I do both skype and live coaching, depending on what the person needs. Because of my hands-on approach, I don't accept everyone; instead I first make sure we'd be a good fit and you have the right attitude about training. So if you'd like to learn more, send me an email to Psych@ModernFlirting.com describing your situation, and what you'd like to accomplish. If accepted, we can then sit down and talk about creating a new you.

With that said, I'm confident you now have the tools to go out there to approach your dream girl tonight. I want to thank you for taking the time to read this and hopefully, putting it to good use. No matter what you ultimately decide to do though, never stop learning.

"Develop a passion for learning. If you do, you will never cease to grow."

- Anthony J. D'Angelo

About The Author

Jared "Psych" Laurence is an international motivational speaker, as well as a globally recognized Lifestyle Consultant and Dating Specialist.

Over the past 12+ years Psych has been voted the best new dating coach, taught over 10,000 students around the world, and is credited with countless relationships and marriages.

Using classically trained counseling and cutting-edge techniques, he has helped all types of clients. This includes professional multimillionaires, programmers, finance guys, and even college students.

No stranger to helping those in distress, after volunteering at a suicide and crisis hotline center, he found his calling in coaching and mentorship.

He's been featured in seminars and popular media including:

- MTV's "Made"
- Oxygen's "Bad Girls Club"
- A&E Documentary "Born This Way
- "The Great Love Debate"
- "The 21 Convention Men's Conference"
- "World Dating Coach Summit"
- ABC's "Nightline"
- And repeated guest on the radio show "Waking up in Vegas."